HEALTY HABITS
SHARP MIND

KEYS TO INCREASE MEMORY AND CREATIVITY IN NATURAL WAYS

Dr. Annex Harp

JOLPIC PUBLICATION

HEALTHY HABITS SHARP MIND

First Edition: May, 2019

JOLPIC PUBLICATION

ISBN: 9781098965303

E-book also available

Dedicated to The Creator

Preface

This book is meant for those people who need a sharp and healthy brain with an enormous power of photographic memory. Your brain is the gift of god and driving you every moment. Your mind is a free bird and it diverts from its way and as a result, the mind becomes weak. Then you start to forget information, your creative ideas get lost and you fail to do simple everyday tasks.

This book tells you how to manipulate your brain by following some simple tricks. You can do anything with your brain, your brain is not weak, you have suppressed your brain power with your daily habits. Change your life with the help of this book and get a healthy brain which does not get old. Following these techniques get refreshed young brain even if you reached at seventy.

And finally, don't judge this book by its small size. This book can be an atom bomb for you.

Author

TABLE OF CONTENT

1

Good Workout

Your brain is made of millions of neural pathways and they developed a circuit to give you consciousness. Your brain is said to be healthy when it can recall information quickly, solve mathematical problems, and perform typical tasks with a least of mental effort. Your brain is similar to a computer which has both a RAM and ROM. Your memory is decided by your brain's ROM and intelligence is a measure of your brain's RAM. Your brain's ROM collects information every day and having it you can recall things, remember old friend names and their phone numbers etc. whereas your brain's RAM helps you to solve problems quickly, you can take efficient decisions in your way, you can create new ideas like a scientist. Both the RAM and ROM of your brain are necessary to lead a healthy lifestyle.

From your childhood to adulthood brain has gone through a process of development and at a certain age, its development stops. Then, reaching a certain age at your thirties, it passes through a process of decaying. Your brain is going older and it power will diminish very slowly without your notice. When you reach your old age, it becomes difficult to remember trivial things, you cannot concentrate to your work and life becomes tougher.

But there are several ways which can protect your brain from ageing. But remember, from your childhood to adulthood, it is necessary to nourish your brain very effective way, so that it can reach its highest peak of its development. If you torture your brain from the very beginning, you can expect that it will betray you at your old age. So, be careful at early stage.

Your brain needs stimulations. Working out effective and healthy exercises for your brain are most effective way for your brain's growth and development. Start at your early age so that your brain can get its ultimate power and a good healthy brain decay very slowly. And continuation of these exercises for your brain provide you an immortal brain which will not lose its power over time.

Power of your brain behaves line your muscle strength, more you use, it gets stronger. Without us, it gets dull. The more you work out your brain, the better you will be able to remember information. But not all work outs are the same. Different activities for your brain needs different exercises. To regrow your losing memory, you can do following exercise in your daily routine. How much effective these are beyond your imaginations.

Start New Activities:

You have a busy schedule in your day job. You are very busy due to some workloads from your office or from your home. But, you need to take out times for you own, because you are not able to get a healthy brain with pressure, you must require a relaxing mental condition which will be very effective to increase both your memory and intelligence. It is necessary, in that extra time you have to do something new. Some ideas are given here and those are scientifically proven.

1) Start to learn a new language

Maybe you are very good at your mother tongue or you already know a few more other languages and you also have good vocabulary in those. But it may not be enough for your brain. Try to learn one more languages and grow your vocabulary in it as well. It can efficiently boost your brain day by day. A fresh brain can learn a language very quickly. Researchers say, age seven is the best age for learning new language and grow vocabulary. But remember, you are not a seven-year boy. You are much older, so you will take more times to learn it than a seven years old boy. While you are learning, your brain is getting stronger and refresh, in other words, it is tending to become a seven-year boy's brain.

I can suggest one thing more. Choose a language which is much different from your mother tongue. Then you can learn a better way, you are learning to construct sentences with a new grammar which effectively regrow your brain. Moreover, new alphabets and vocabulary simultaneously improve your memory.

When you become ready, start to use it. Do conversation with new people of other country with that language. Many communicative medias are available today to make new friends from other countries. So start from today.

2) __Learn a musical instrument__

Music is one kind of food for your brain. Music can make you happy and give a boost to your brain. However, playing a music yourself is far way better than listening to it. When you are playing a musical instrument with remembering notes, your brain is getting a tingling and some neurons getting its more lifetime to die.

Learning a music instrument becomes lot easier than ten years ago. Now you can learn it yourself. There are many tutorial site in internet where you can find your full course.

3) __Write a book__

Writing a book is a good idea and it is challenging too. When you start to write, your imaginative power increases, you make stories and thus you are continuously using your brain and preventing its ageing process. There are several ways to self-publish your book and you can earn money as well.

4) __Do painting__

Painting is another way to make your brain busy and passing your leisure in an active way. Painting is as useful as writing a book. It increases your imaginative power which is good for your brain health.

5) __Learn Cooking__

Join cooking courses, it may help you to improve your memory. Just remember ingredients and try the recipe yourself later.

6) __Learn new brain games__

Learn some indoor games which uses brain to play, for example, chess, card games, Chinese checker etc. There are many games available in other countries. Search internet and find out those games. Then, start to learn and play with your friends.

Do mental exercises

These methods are very easy to maintain in your daily routine, even you can apply it when you are busy at your work. So, you have to definitely apply these methods to increase your brain power.

1) Remember list

It did happen some times that someone handed over you a list of things to bring those when you were going for shopping. The best idea is, do not take the list and remember it into your head so that you can easily fetch those things by recalling. It is an effective idea for increasing your memory power.

2) Do Calculations

When you are at shopping, you add up prices of things by taking a paper and pen or using a calculator. But you can do the sum using your mind. Next time, do not use pen and paper or calculator, use your own head.

3) Draw maps

Draw a map of your recently visited places from your memory. It is a test for your brain health as well as good for your brain health.

4) Read books

Reading a story book or novel is best idea to resist cognitive decline. When you read a story, sometimes you make characters alive unconsciously, you imagine new places from the stories, you make scenes just like you are watching a movie in your head. It gives your brain cells a longer lifetime.

5) Play games

Playing puzzles, chess or playing cards are very effective in delaying ageing process of your brain. Find some partners and play occasionally.

You can also try word games, jumbles and any type of other games in which you continuously use your brain.

6) Solve crossword and Sudoku in your daily newspaper

Crossword puzzles help you to test your memory power as well it increases your vocabulary. On the other hand, Sudoku puzzles are effective to grow your intelligence and boost you to solve problems faster.

7) Solve 10th standard math

It sounds funny but as effective as a giant. Open your childhood books one more time. Start to solve arithmetic, algebra and geometry problems again. It is one of the fastest methods to boost your brain. You can see the difference within one week.

2

Physical Exercises

All parts of your body are connected together. You cannot imagine your head without your body or vice versa. Mental exercise is very much required for your brain health but physical exercises are equally important to maintain your brain stay sharp. Maintaining regularity in physical exercises increases oxygen to your brain and keep you away from risks of disorder like memory loss. It reduces the chances of cardiovascular diseases and maintain a low sugar level in your blood. These diseases are responsible for memory loss and reduces the capabilities of your brain. Moreover, physical exercises increase the secretion of required chemicals and hormones inside your brain.

And most importantly exercise can increase plasticity of brain cells and boost their growth factor which stimulate the new neural connectivity.

But all physical exercises are not good for all. A sixty years old man may not run as fast as teenagers. So, we have to modify some exercises according to ages. In this chapter, some exercises have been discussed which are good for all ages. Maintain a daily routine for those and get a healthy brain.

1) Getting up from bed

Do you feel an unnecessary drowsiness when you rise from bed in morning? If it last longer, you need to do some physical activity after getting up and see the changes in a few days.

After opening your eyes in morning, take a deep breath and breath out for five minutes. It provides you required oxygen to your head and you will feel normal within a few minutes. Do not think anything during this exercise, keep a refreshed mind. After that walk slowly but steadily on your floor for 3 – 5 minutes. It will reduce your drowsiness and you will get a charm to start a new day.

2) Jogging

You can do jogging in morning or evening time, but do not do with stomach full. It is a process of running in slowly and leisurely manner. Do for 30 – 40 minutes according to your health and age.

Find a few friends if you want some company.

3) Walking

Always walk, walking is the best exercise. It does not need any time or place; you can walk whenever you want. But maintain some rule while you are walking. Keep a good speed than normal and keep your body completely straight.

Some people avoid walk and ride a car for a few kilometer distance. It is bad for their health. You can easily cross that distance within 30 minutes and it good for blood circulation in your brain.

4) Cycling

Cycling is another good exercise but less efficient than walking. But you require both for maintaining a good brain health. Twenty minutes cycling is enough for a day.

5) Jumping

Jumping is advised when you are not getting proper place for jogging. You can do it on the floor at your room or on your garden. Gently jump 20 – 30 times, then take a break for 5-10 minutes, and again continue. Repeat the cycle for 30 – 40 minutes daily.

6) Breathing

It is not a kind of physical exercise but very efficient method to deliver oxygen in your head. Take a deep breath and slowly breath out. Continue it for 5 minutes. Then take rest for 10 minutes. Continue for 30 minutes. It gives a quick boost to your brain.

All these exercises may not enough for your physical health but these are good for maintaining a healthy brain.

3

Sleeping Rules

Everyone sleeps regularly and you also. A good amount of sleep is most required thing to get a healthy brain. But there are huge differences between a good sleep and bad sleep. Most of the people do not have the idea of how to sleep perfectly. Some people feel drowsiness for entire day due to an incomplete sleeping practices. And also some people cannot sleep quickly on bed thus late night sleeping is silently killing their brain cells without informing them. Adults need to sleep for 7.5 to 9 hours in order to avoid sleep deprivation. A good sleeping practice can improve memory, problem solving abilities, skills of critical thinking and creativities day by day. Research shows that memory enhancement occurs at the deepest stage of your sleeping. So, you need to maintain some rules for your efficient sleeping activity.

1) Sleeping schedule

Maintain a tight schedule for your sleep. Do not deviate from that. Usually 11 PM to 7 PM is best for you in order to maintain the 8 hours' rule. Try not to break your routine, even on weekends and holidays.

2) Sleeping bed

For a comfortable sleeping activity, choose a clean bed which should be not too much soft or too much hard. Bedsheet should be made of 100% cotton. Light colored bedsheets are good for sleeping since those are poor heat absorber.

3) Sleeping place

Your room should be clean. Room should be odorless and filled with enough oxygen. An air conditioning system will be good for you with a thin blanket. Curtains should be dark in color to avoid morning sunlight. Room should be completely dark and free of any sound to get an undisturbed deep sleep.

4) Don't

Switch off your mobile phones one hour before your sleeping. Recent research shows that any electromagnetic radiations on your surrounding can disturb your sleep. Switch off also television, radio, Wi-Fi, or any other electronic devices before sleeping.

5) Do not use alarm

A sudden tweak from your deep sleep condition is as harmful as sleeplessness. So, do not use alarm on your table clock. Your brain already has a precise watch to make you awake. If you maintain a same sleeping schedule regularly, you will be able to rise from bed at a particular time.

6) Sleep quickly

It becomes a major problem in our stressful life that we are not able to sleep too quickly after catching our bed. Some people remain awake hour after hour and their brain is damaging day by day. You can follow some tips in order to sleep quickly.

- Do a 30 minutes physical exercise before sleeping.
- Do not use mobile or television before your sleeping.
- You can read a short story book on your bed. It will ultimately make you asleep.
- Sleep under complete darkness.
- Do breathing exercise laying on bed.
- Remove all of your thoughts while sleeping.
- Concentrate your mind on the middle of middle of your head.
- Do not drink coffee or tea before sleeping.
- Do not smoke cigarette or drink alcohol.

7) Day nap

A day nap can improve your brain power. After a stressful work, take a quick nap, it will warm up to your brain and increase your creativity power.

8) Meditation

Meditation is good for perfect sleep. You can also try meditation before bed.

4

Dos and Don'ts

Getting a healthy brain is not an easy task to do or it is as easy as beyond your imagination. It needs prolonged practice including lifestyle changing, dealing with other people, training your brain and other multiple tricks. If you can manage to do for a long period of time, your brain will be a slave near you. You will become a person of influence. Then you will be able to train others. Follow some simple rules and make the changes in your life.

You are thinking something in every moment in your life. You cannot live without any thought. Your thought can be good or bad for your brain health thus you have to control your thought with a trained mind. If any bad thought captures your brain for a prolonged period of time, no doubt, it will definitely damage your brain cells and one time will come when you will not get escape from such unavoidable situation.

Every bad habit is also responsible to reduce your mind power, so you need get rid from those habits also. I shall try to cover up almost all the situations that you will probably face in your life and advise you to reduce all the bad habits that you have in your daily life.

1) Do not watch TV (Don't)

Many habits are associated with your life that these have long term effect in your future. Watching television is one of those. Probably you have noticed when you watched television for a prolonged period time and tried to do a vital work after that, your work has gone wrong. While you are watching TV, it is making tired your brain, as a result, when you try to concentrate on your study or on other job, your brain fails to do. Your study or job remains incomplete.

If you routinely watch television, you get addicted, and after a long period of time your brain cells start to die. When you reach at 60 – 70 age, you fail to remember trivial things. So, my suggestion is that try to avoid television as far as possible.

2) Do not play video games (Don't)
Video games are curse of our technological achievements. You must have an android phone and downloaded several games from the play-store to play every day. Those games in your computer or mobile phone affect your brain two times faster rate than television. Delete those games from today because you will get effect of those after 30 – 40 years when you will have no options to get back a healthy brain.

3) Avoid negative people (Don't)
Some people always think negative and try to implement negative thinking in your mind.

Always avoid those people. Negative talk or negative thought always gives you stress and damage your brain. Sometimes it can make you depressed. So, do not think negative or do not let other people to make you think negative.

4) Do not think much (Don't)

Do not think about anything for a long period of time. The thoughts will make you unhappy. Even do not think about any happy moment too. Sometimes, a thought can lead you to next day and then day after day. So, do not think about anything for a long time even the thought is being positive. Just mumble *hakuna matata*.

5) Addict to books (Dos)

Only one addiction in this entire world is good that is reading books. Spend your leisure time with books. Read any type of books that you prefer to read and gain knowledge. Book can nourish your damaged brain cell and keep them active.

6) Keep yourself busy (Dos)

Always try to stay busy doing any constructive work. Choose a topic in which you are passionate about and concentrate on that. A busy mind cannot think negative or cannot be depressed.

7) Do not get addicted (Don't)

Do not get addicted to anything bad or get addicted towards any people. Addiction to anything or anyone always resist you from your day job. You become divert from your routine and waste your time. Addiction towards anything is equally harmful, it may be TV shows, movies, games, your lover, your child, your wife etcetera. So stay away from addiction. But, it does not mean you are supposed ignore any particular person in order to avoid him/her.

8) Do not fight with other (Don't)

Do not quarrel or argue with other people. If you are feeling, you are right and another person are wrong, do not argue with him/her.

Stay calm and try to solve the problem with discussions. Avoid talking with loud voice; it is indeed harmful for your brain. Remember, you cannot change other peoples' mind with your loud voice. Always avoid those circumstances which will make you angry. It will be better to retreat away.

9) Do not recall past or think about the future (Don't)

Thinking about past incident will make you weak and ultimately you will be depressed. Do not think about past incident anymore. You cannot get back past time. Same is true for the future, do not think about the future also, future can be bad or good. It is not in your hand. So, why are you thinking?

Concentrate only to the present. Give your hundred percent to make your future good (it is your expectation not thinking). Definitely God will give you greatest reward later.

10)   Avoid gossips (Don't)

Do not talk about other peoples' activities to anyone. All people have their personal lives. You have no right to interfere.

11)   Do not hate others

It may possible that someone did bad to you in past. Try to forgive him/her because keeping a thought of revenge in your mind is slowly destroying your brain. A revengeful mind can make you psychological patient in future. It will do nothing bad for the said person but it is very bad for your mental health.

12)   Always try to stay happy

Nothing is precious than a happy mind. Do some job which will make you happy. It can be writing books, painting, singing etcetera.

13)   Travelling

When you feel depressed for any reason, do not worry, pack your bags and plan a trip for a week. It works like magic. Your sadness will vanish within a few days. Of course, take you're a few friends in that trip.

5

Social Interactions

The secret of having a healthy brain is living a happy life. And the primary rule for happy life is never stay alone. However, sometimes passing time only with yourself is important but not always. Maybe you are a busy person or you have enough time to spend but remember interaction with other people is very important in order to live a happy life. When you are talking with your friend, some chemicals in your brain make your neurons healthy, so the brain gets more longevity. researchers found that an active social life had the slowest rate of memory decline.

Some suggestions are given below.

1) Spend time with friends

Make some times for your friends and family at least once in a week. Many studies show that a life full of friends and fun comes with cognitive benefits. But do not always think of serious talk with them, have some fun, make laughter. More you laugh, more you gain. Watch a funny movie. Go to a restaurant and eat delicious dishes. Do whatever you want for your fun and enjoyment.

2) Keep good relation with your neighborhoods

Yes. It is important. Keeping a good relation with neighbors will make your home a place of happy living. They will also help you when you fall in some danger. You can also spend time with them that will make your brain healthier.

3) Talk with people

Always talk with other people when you get some chances. For example, when you are feeling tired in your office in the mid of a tough work, stop your work for ten minutes and talk with your colleague in your surroundings. You will feel the difference instantly, your mind will be refreshed and deliver you some extra energy to complete your left work. It is very good for your mental health.

4) Talk to stranger

Do not stay alone in a long journey, talk with people besides you. Continuing a 3-4 hours journey without any activity will make you bored, and when you feel bored, amount of chemical secretion in your brain suddenly stops. So, try to talk with stranger when possible but do not take them seriously in your life.

5) Keep a pet

Do you like animals like dog or cat? Buy one. Spending time with them increase hormonal secretion in your head and your brain gets stronger. Believe me, they can be a best friend in your life.

6) Join a club

A club is the best place to interact with other people. It will also help you increase your physical activity. Join a club today.

7) Use your phone

You can talk with old friend with your mobile phone but do not habituate with it. Regular talking for a long time with your phone can damage your brain in the near future.

8) Do not type chat

There are several social media available on internet or android phones where you can chat with someone by typing. But avoid it as far as you can, it can be bad for your brain. Type chatting is time consuming process and you are giving pressure to your brain while doing it. Always try to interact with people by face to face rather in a virtual world.

9) Healthy relationship

Always try to maintain a healthy relationship with your partner. It is necessity for your brain.

10) Do not find wrong friends

Avoid those people who bore you or you unlike them (no matter they are good or bad). But it is okay when they are in a group of other good friends.

6

Stress

Your brain's worst enemy is stress. Nothing can save your brain from memory loss if you have a stressful mind. Chronic stress destroys brain cells and damages the hippocampus. Hippocampus is associated with formation and recovery of memories. Research showed a stressful mind loses memory in faster rate than a happy brain. Stress can also lead you to depression and anxiety, so get rid from stress. Here are some basic rules in order to manage your stress.

1) Limit your expectation

You cannot be another Bill Gates. I am not discouraging you with that sentence but accept the truth. You are earning money for a happy life but do not try to destroy your happiness for bringing more money. Human life is short and after a certain age you will feel too much money is meaning less in your life, and all will be left back after your death. So, try to live a happy life with your limited amount of money. Give your effort only to your work and do not think that you are working because of getting money, you are working because you simply love it.

2) Find an appropriate job

Do not continue a job which is not bring happiness for you, you are doing because you are pressurized to do so. Suppose you are working in police department but you are passionate about to become a teacher, believe me, one time will come when you feel stress in your life. Take decision beforehand, find an appropriate job for you even if the salary is lesser.

3) Take some break

Do not continue a task for a long period of time, take a break for 10 -20 minutes at a certain interval of time. It will refresh your mind.

4) Avoid multitasking

Concentrate on a single work at a time. Do not try to do two or more tasks together. It will reduce the efficiency for both the tasks, moreover, prolonged practice of multitasking may cause anxiety to your mental health.

5) Plan for the next day

It is one of the best practices in order to manage your time and also good for your mental health. Use a pocket diary and note what you planned to do for tomorrow. Also make a routine for the next day. It a target for you what you are going to do in the next day. In a few days you will notice that efficiency of your work has increased several time faster than before. Doing work in a faster rate will give you mental satisfaction.

6) Quit tobacco and alcohol

Tobacco and alcohol is the definite reason for depression and anxiety. These create chemical imbalances inside your brain, as a result, you lose your memory over time. Moreover, these can result other health deceases which will indirectly affect your brain.

7) Reduce stresses by other way

I have already discussed these techniques. These have instant abilities to reduce stress.

- Travelling
- Hangout with friends
- Your hobbies, such as singing, dancing, painting etc.

8) Spend time with children

Spend your time with children and interact them pretending yourself as a small child. It will help you to reduce stress.

9) Meditation

Meditation has several other health benefit including your brain's health. Researches show that meditation helps to improve many different types of health conditions, including depression, anxiety, chronic pain, diabetes, and high blood pressure. Meditation also improve focus, concentration, creativity, memory, learning and reasoning skills. No other activity can beat meditation.

Meditation shows its magic by changing your actual brain. Practicing meditations have more activity in the left prefrontal cortex which controls your feelings of joy and self-control. Meditation also increases the thickness of the cerebral cortex and creates more connections between brain cells – which increases mental sharpness and memory ability.

10) Balance work and leisure time

It is very important to maintain a healthy balance between your work and leisure time. Doing work by all over the day can lead you to severe anxiety and depression. Separate out some amount of time from your daily routine only for your own.

11) Express your feelings to others

Do not bottle up your feelings of joy or sorrow inside your head rather express it someone (but not to everyone). When you are hiding your anger or sorrow, your brain is putting into pressure and it will make you depressed over time. When you talk about it with someone, you will feel free and your stress will be reduced to some extent.

7

Laugh, Laugh and Laugh!

Probably you have heard the proverb "LAUGHTER IS THE BEST MEDICINE" and indeed that proverb is correct. When you laugh, most of the areas of your brain gets stimulations with secretion of hormones that makes your brain perfectly chemically balanced. Other happy emotions work on your brain at certain region which is far less effective than a laugh. Do anything for your laugh, watch a funny movie, make fun, anything that you can. If you lead a life with filled of laughter, make sure it has a prolonged effect in your life. It can delay your ageing process, keep you away from Alzheimer's, increase your memory and creativity, and above all it can give you a physically fit body.

You have to find out laugh in your own way but I can help you to provide some idea which will help you in the way of finding out laughter.

1) Listening to jokes

Listen to jokes whenever you get the chances. It is far better when someone tells you a jokes instead you read it in any book or newspaper. When someone tells you a jokes you try to laugh even if it is not so much funny because you always try to encourage the person with a laugh. Your laugh is important, no matter how much fun you have got. Listening to a hilarious jokes activates areas of the brain vital to learning and creativity.

You can also buy some hilarious books for enjoyment but those are less effective if you do not laugh by those.

2) Watch funny TV shows and movies

Watching a funny TV shows or movies (TV is harmful to you but not this time) is equally effective as listening to a joke. Take some other persons for company, laugh may not come when you are alone.

3) Laugh at yourself

Share your funny and embarrassing moments with your friends and laugh. Laugh is very much contagious, when your friends start to laugh, you will follow them too.

4) Search for laughter

When you hear some laughter, move toward it. People are very happy to share something funny because it gives them an opportunity to laugh again. When you hear laughter, try to join in.

5) Make friendship with funny people

Some people find laugh in everyday events. They are hilarious and fun loving. They create fun, even in very saddest moment. Spend time with those playful people, make them friends. Don't forget, laughter is contagious.

6) Create a funny surroundings

This method is less effective but sometime work. Paste some funny poster at your home. Change your computer desktop and mobile screen with funny pictures. Put some funny toys or figures here and there at your home. These will make your life more delightful.

7) Do fun with children

Children are fun loving, they can take life lightly. Spend some time with them and act like childish. You will find some laughter with those happiest children.

8

Diet

Your every effort can go in vain if you do not maintain a healthy diet. Just like your body, your brain also need fuel to run properly. A healthy diet is required for brain cell growth and synthesizing required hormones for your brain. A diet containing fruits and vegetables can improve your memory a way faster than normal. Moreover, a healthy diet will keep away you from doctors and it has enormous health benefits. The following nutritional tips will help you to boost your brainpower and reduce risk of dementia.

1) Fishes

Omega-3 fatty acid is primarily important for your brain health. Oily fishes are excellent sources for omega-3 fatty acids. Salmon, tuna, halibut, trout, mackerel, sardines, oyster and herring etc. fishes are rich sources of that.

2) Vegetables

Besides fishes, some vegetables also have omega-3. seaweed, walnuts, ground flaxseed, flaxseed oil, winter squash, kidney and pinto beans, spinach, broccoli, pumpkin seeds, and soybeans are the non-fish sources.

3) Fruit and vegetables

Eat more fruit and vegetables. These will produce enough antioxidants, which will protect your brain cells from damage. Colored fruits and vegetables are particularly good antioxidant sources.

4) Limit saturated fats

Saturated fats can lead you to high risk of memory loss and reduce concentration ability. Avoid saturated fat containing food such as red meat, whole milk, butter, cheese, cream, and ice cream.

5) Green tea

Increase intake of green tea. Green tea contains polyphenols which is powerful antioxidants efficient to protect free radicals formation (that can damage brain cells). Researchers found regular consumption of green tea may enhance memory and slow down brain ageing process.

6) Drink wine

Alcohol generally harmful to your brain since alcohol kills brain cells. But a limited amount of drinking wine is actually beneficial to your brain health, it increases your memory power. Red wine is the best option for you, drink one or two cup twice in a week. It is rich in resveratrol that increases blood circulation in the brain and reduces the risk of dementia.

7) Drink fruit juice

Grape juice, cranberry juice, and berries are the rich sources of resveratrol. You can try it instead of wine.

8) Quit addictive stimulators

Quit smoking cigarettes and excessive alcohol or any other types of addictive substances. Those are as harmful as poison for your brain.

9) Avoid toxic metal

Ground water in some places contains toxic metals such as aluminum and copper. Do not drink those water without testing it.

9

Check Health

D o you feel that your memory is suddenly dropped in recent days? You are feeling difficulty to recall your favorite actors name or your friends' name. Even you are putting wrong pin for your ATM card to purchase things or forgetting your mail password. You are continuously missing things at your home. Be sure, those are results of health or lifestyle problems. Not only dementia or Alzheimer's is related to your memory drop, there may have other health problems that is interfering to your memory. Visit a doctor and identify and treat those health problems.

1) Heart disease

Cardiovascular disease and its risk factors for example high cholesterol and high blood pressure may responsible for your memory loss.

2) Diabetes

People with high sugar level in their blood are likely to be a cause of forgetfulness.

3) Hormonal disorder

After menopause, women often experience memory problems due to their estrogen decrease. Whereas for men, low testosterone level can create the same issues. Thyroid imbalances can also cause forgetfulness, lazy thinking, or confusion.

4) Medicines

Cold and allergy medicines, sleeping pills, and antidepressant drugs may be a cause of memory loss. Talk to your doctor about their side effects and take proper action to reduce their effects.

It will be better to avoid those medicines as far as you can. If you follow a perfectly balanced life you will have no need of antidepressants or sleeping pill. An ordinary allergy or cold can be cured within a few days so do not take medicines for an ordinary viral flu.

5) Depression

Mental sluggishness, difficulty in concentration, and forgetfulness are common symptoms of depression. A depression sometimes can be wrongly treated for dementia since their symptoms are almost same.

But there is a good news. When the depression is treated accurately, memory returns to normal.

6) Toxicity or allergy

Sometimes toxicity or allergic effect for a particular food can cause a severe drop in memory. Identify and reject those foods.

10

Practical Methods

This is the final chapter in this book and it the most vital chapter. Maybe someone has an extraordinary memory, however, memory has its limits. No one can hold in his brain an uncountable numbers of data. But sometimes there are many information that we have to put them in our head. Ultimately we fail to remember those and fall in embarrassed situations in our life. Here are some very basic but effective techniques that will help you most of the time, I hope.

1) Pay attention

Always pay 100% attention when you are learning something new. Your brain needs 8 seconds to consume an information into your memory. If you become easily distracted while learning, you may not recall it on your crucial moment and it is equal to – you never learned that lesson. Thus, paying concentration is vital technique for your learning process.

If you distracted easily by any noise or disturbance, find a quiet and calm place where you can pay attention without any interruption.

2) Use your all senses

Try to gather all the information with your five sense organs, eyes, nose, ear, skin and tongue when possible. Suppose you in a restaurant, you listen name of a new food, you can better remember the name if you would taste it. You can easily remember a poem if you read out loud.

3) Write down

If you want to remember any paragraph from a book, write it down in your notebook several times without seeing it.

4) Make a gist

Note down useful points from a chapter of a book without remembering the whole book. For example, you can note down only bold points of this book so that you can remember the whole book at once.

5) Relate information from previous learning

Try to relate information from your previous learning. Suppose you want to remember a person's name, ask him his address; if you recall his city of living (it is familiar to you), you can easily recall his name too.

6) Focus on the concept rather whole thing

For complex material such as physics or chemistry, emphasis on understanding the basic ideas rather than memorizing all details.

7) Explain to someone

Explain to someone what you have just learned, it will help you to memorize and consume your lessons.

8) Quick rehearse

Within five minutes after learning o through the pages of your notebook and recapitulate it at least two times. It will help you to remember quickly.

9) Mnemonics

Mnemonics is a special kind of technique that is often used to remember things. You can also make new mnemonics in your own techniques. It demands some detailed discussion to understand the idea.

Mnemonics

Visual image

Create a visual image in your mind to memorize a name. Suppose you want to memorize a name "Rosa Hills", just make a picture of rose and mountains subsequently, you will recall her name easily.

Acrostic (or sentence)

Make a sentence in which the first letter of each word is initial of what you want to remember. For example, "Memory Needs Every Method Of Nurturing Its Capacity" is a mnemonic for memorize the spelling 'mnemonic.'

Acronym

An acronym is a word that is made up by taking the first letters of all the words you need to remember and creating a new word out of them.

For example, "BODMAS" is an acronym for doing long arithmetic calculation. BODMAS is an acronym and it stands for Bracket, Of, Division, Multiplication, Addition and Subtraction.

Rhymes and alliteration

Rhymes, alliteration (a repeating sound or syllable), are the method to remember facts and figures. Example: The rhyme "Thirty days hath September, April, June, and November" to remember the months of the year with only 30 days in them.

Chunking

Chunking is associated with breaking a long list of numbers or other types of information into smaller parts. Example: A 10-digit phone number can be remembered by breaking it into three sets of numbers.

Method of loci

Imagine placing items in specific locations in your familiar room or building if you want to remember them in a sequential order.

Example: For a shopping list

Banana

Puddle

Eggs

bread

imagine bananas in the entryway to your home, a puddle of milk in the middle of the sofa, eggs going up the stairs, and bread on your bed.

*All the above **'mnemonic'** methods are very effective in order to remember information. I hope, you could understand the basic idea of mnemonic and you will make some new.*